Diabetes:
An Emotional Journey

by
Renea Jo Zosel

Illustrations
by
Jeanne Young

Published by
Zay Publishing and Consulting Company.
27414 236th Place SE
Maple Valley, WA 98038
206-498-5055
www.zaypub.com

Library of Congress Control Number: 2003111050
ISBN: 0-9743431-0-2
Printed and handmade in The United States of America

DISCLAIMER

This book does not intend to give medical advice. Always contact your doctor or health care provider for assistance. The experiences in this book are not intended to be a substitute for consulting with a health care provider. All issues regarding your health, medications, and use of medical devices require medical supervision.

I have put together this book after four years of writing finally found their way into a computer. This book is for families affected by diabetes. As you read through this journey, you will know that you are not alone with your desperation, anger, sorrow, fear, love, courage and resolve.

This book is for all sisters, brothers, aunts, uncles, in-laws, parents and grand parents. It is for all of our health care providers, teachers, volunteers, politicians and social workers. This book is also for my family, my dear friends who sometimes wish they didn't understand and for those who want to understand.

I hope that as you read this book, you will be able to enter in for a moment to this emotional journey. I want you to understand this ride like you never have before so that you can offer support like you never have before. If the terms and definitions that I use are intimidating, please refer to the definitions in the back of this book.

Finally, when you do understand, if but for a minute, show your support. Learn how to manage diabetes, offer respite care, house clean, go out for coffee, go to the park, join the Juvenile Diabetes Research Foundation, or the American Diabetes Association, fund- raise, care, pray... You will be giving more than you can imagine.

This is a never-ending, scenery-changing ride and we all need supporters.

Renea Jo Zosel

CONTENTS

I do not have diabetes living in my body...
I do not experience the physical effects of tumultuous blood sugars.
I do not face endless finger pokes, site changes and doctors visits.

I do have diabetes living in my head...
I do feel the anguish as I watch my daughter bounce from low to high.
I do deliver the endless finger pokes and site changes and doctors visits.

I live diabetes...
While my daughter who has diabetes, just lives.
She knows no other way of life.

I did.
I do.
I always will.

THE BEGINNING

Fall 1999

As we began to potty train our daughter Elizabeth, we became acutely aware that all was not well. She drank at least 10 sippy cups of water a day. She would soak a brand new diaper and then drip through onto the floor in minutes. I was vaguely aware of the symptoms of diabetes because my cousin has had it for years. After a worried call to my mother, we made an immediate appointment with our pediatrician. The visit was the beginning of the end of normal as we knew it.

Along with excessive thirst and frequent urination, there is rapid weight loss, lethargy and ultimately a ketoacidosis-induced coma. Elizabeth didn't experience these other symptoms because we had caught the autoimmune disease, juvenile diabetes (also called diabetes mellitus or type I diabetes) quickly.

We spent 3 days in the hospital, learning a new way of life and unlearning all the stereotypes we held about diabetes.

We learned that she will not outgrow diabetes. She will grow up, but juvenile diabetes will always be with her. Yes, she can have sugar if it is counted in her daily diet plan. No, she won't die young, but without insulin she will die. Her body does not produce insulin, and a pill won't help. Yes, she can have children. Yes, she can do whatever she wants. Yes, she will live a full life. This is not the end of the world, it just feels like it.

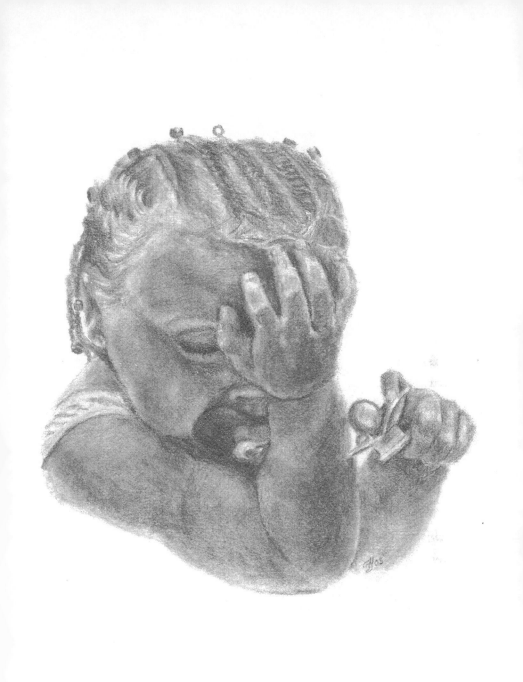

It crept in so slowly
little as it was

We didn't notice
until water flooded
the place too many times.

It took her away so quickly
big as she was

We didn't realize
how our lives would change.

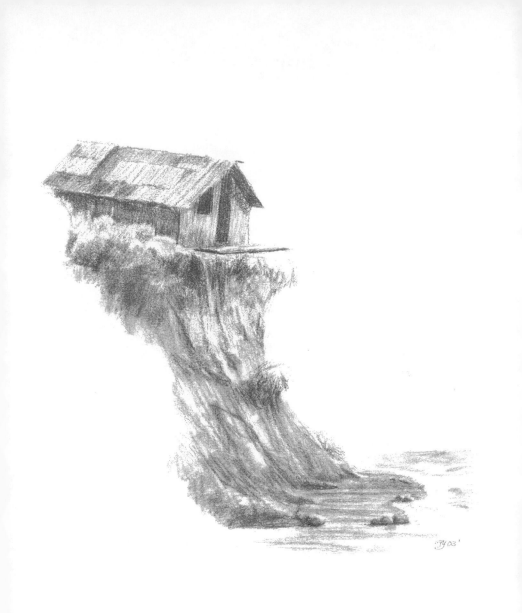

DESPERATION

She is my daughter
My blood, my flesh
My creation.

I am her mother
Her protection, her balance
Her stability.

I cannot control,
make normal,
get rid of
this thing possessing my baby.

I cannot make it go away.
I am supposed to.
I am her mother.

She has diabetes.
I cannot cure her.

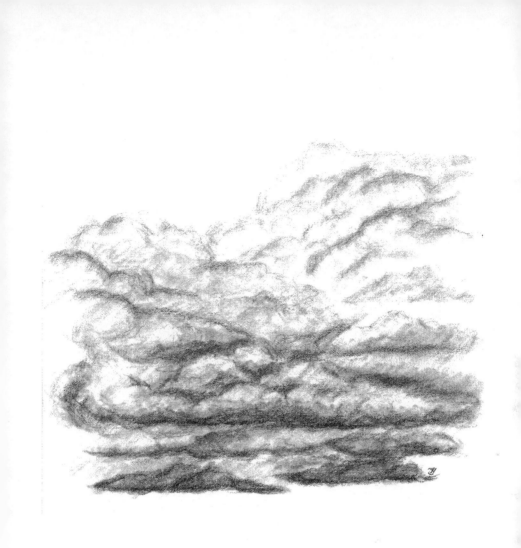

ANGER

It floods my being
wrecking my soul
forcing me to look
into the depths of hatred.

It leaves my being
erasing my past
prying open my mind
forcing me to love her pain.

It takes control
controls my breath
leaves me speechless
out of control
crying, praying.

It has my baby
flooding her being
tearing through her veins
wrecking her body
begging me to control it.

I try, try, try
TRY to control it
It scares me.
I hate it.

In amazement I watch as my emotions fluctuate.

Anger:
at the disease
at the world for not understanding
at myself for not taking better care of her
and for doing whatever I did to cause this

Happiness:
as I look at my child
receive a hug
plant a kiss
pick dandelions

Hatred:
of the unknown
of the future and what it could bring
of the highs that are wrecking her kidneys, liver, eyes, heart
the lows that are ruining her brain, heart and ....

Love:
love flowing out of me to kiss a finger that I have just made bleed
love overpowering that I keep waking though I am stuck to the bed.

Dear Elizabeth,

I am writing you this letter in hope that my feelings can be set free. You are my daughter, my first born, my baby. I love you more than I can begin to say. You came into my life and with it you brought hopes, dreams and fears.

I want you to have **only** the best. I try so hard to keep your blood sugar under control. I stress and worry about you so much. So much that all that comes across to you, I fear, is a negative, hyper-controlling mother. I get so angry when I can't control the numbers and it comes out at you. I hate diabetes. I hate thinking that someday you could be blind, have a foot or leg amputated, and die because of complications. I hate seeing diabetes in the dreams I have of and for you. I hate it so much that I almost hate you.

But then you smile at me, those beautiful blue eyes sparkling with life and love for me... regardless of the fact that you have diabetes. Diabetes hasn't stopped you from loving me... from laughing... from living.

Elizabeth, I love you so. I am sorry if I do not always show it the way I should. I hope you understand. I love you.

Mom

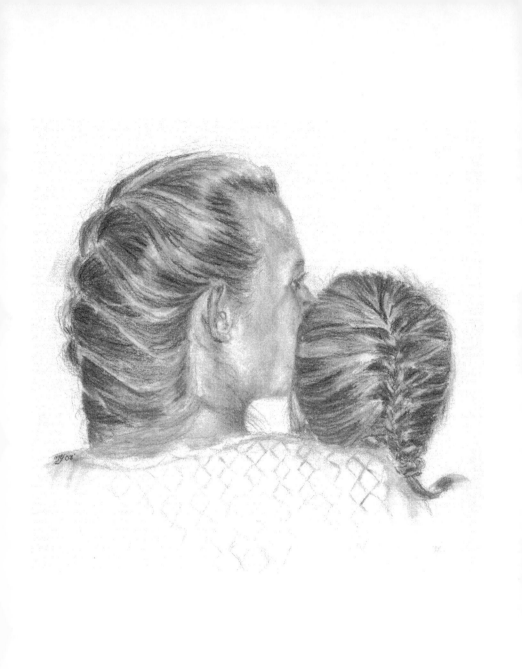

SORROW

Her body is consumed
controlled by a demon
spinning her up into the clouds,
throwing her down
to the ground.
She flies and falls.
Laughing,
joking, screaming,
suffering.

Her mind is consumed
controlled by a thought
killing the demon
forcing it out of her trembling body.
She learns and prays.
Smiling,
comforting, crying,
suffering.

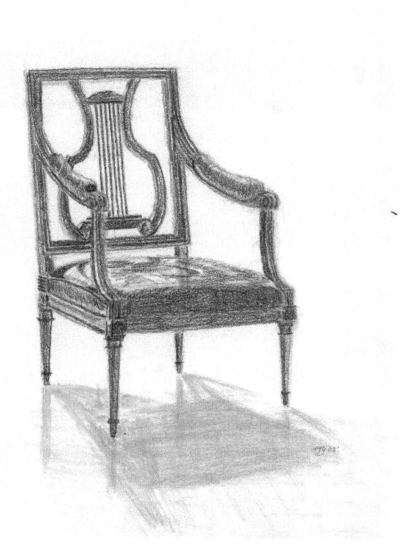

Every Other Day

My heart hurts when I hear and see the pain Elizabeth knows. Some days her cries are barely audible, other days the neighbors come running. She is really so brave, most days she never cries at all even though the memories of pain are always present.

After a bath, as I lotion her hands, I cry silently, although I would like everyone to hear. I hold precious little fingers, poked to calluses. I touch little scars ruptured over and over, tiny holes that don't have a chance to heal because the finger pokes never go away.

We laugh about alligator fingers. I yell inside that alligator skin belongs in the Everglades or on a purse.

At night she falls asleep clutching her bear. I check her blood sugar as she dreams. I see her wince, but she doesn't wake.

I go back to sleep with wet eyes and an ache in my heart.

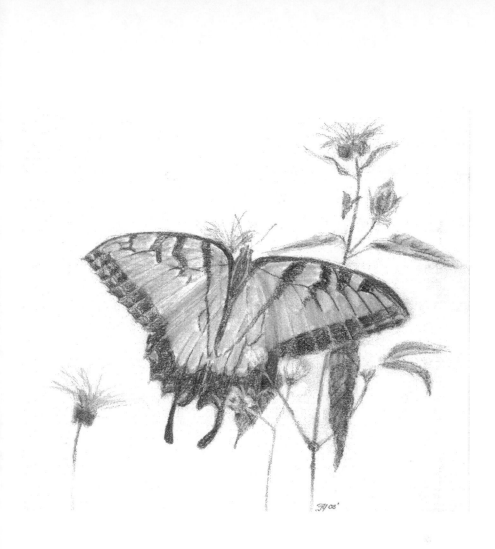

FEAR

Diabetes is scary! There are so many complications that I don't like to think about. I cannot look at my daughter and picture her facing what I know she might, despite our best efforts.

One of the crazy things for us is the possibility of an insulin reaction. Every year that our glucagon expires, I celebrate our good fortune.
Another thing that maybe I fear the most is ketoacidosis. I fear being so far out of control that her body cannot function without hospitalization.

Insulin reactions and ketoacidosis are potentially fatal. I wish they weren't a part of my every day worries.

I fear losing a glucometer, or not bringing it with me in the car even for a quick trip to the store. I fear her pump breaking or malfunctioning or giving too much insulin.

I also fear looking into the eyes of my other children and finding diabetes again.

I am determined though, that these fears will not ruin our lives. They will only make us stronger, and more prepared to live.

First Insulin Reaction

Summer 2001

We slept in late that morning, even baby Katarina, who was usually my alarm clock. The day before had been a glorious summer day: boating, sand castle building, floating in the warm July water. We had experienced just a few low blood sugars, but nothing serious.

9:00 am and I was up, startled by the time and the brightness of the sun. I heard a strange noise, as if someone was gurgling. I knew... I ran... I yelled... I found the glucagon. My daughter, still 3 years old, was completely gone. Foaming saliva was running from her mouth, she was pale, she looked dead. No amount of noise or movement would rouse her. Even after giving her the 'sugar shot' she wasn't with us for 20 minutes, which seemed like a lifetime. I saw her life... and its dreams laying there before me... stretched out... helpless... lifeless. My body ran a marathon by the time she came to.

Not too long after she came back to us, she began to throw up. That is one of the effects of glucagon. I comforted her, rocked her, and cleaned up after her again and again. Then I collapsed from exhaustion.

I would rather have never gone through that experience. I hope that it is not an experience we will have again soon.

We made it, she made it, and SHE WILL MAKE IT!

Ketoacidosis?

Summer 2003

I feel alone tonight. My daughter says this sometimes when she feels funny or doesn't know how to feel and nobody else can understand. Today, I can relate.

My daughter began this morning with a rush to the bathroom where she threw up. We checked for ketones, they were large. We did a poke, 341. We've been higher, so it was nothing to get worked up about, right?
I know what to do for ketones; flush them with fluid and give extra insulin, just get them out of the system. Fine, so we began the 'ketone extraction process'. My husband ran to the store for sugar-free kool-aid. She drank a liter. I checked her every half hour to make sure the insulin was working. The blood sugars barely showed any decline... and I was impatient. Today we were flying to grandma's house. Why did this happen today? We did a site change. We had to make sure she was getting the insulin we were pouring into her.

An hour later she threw up again. We checked ketones again, still large. I knew what was coming but I wanted to avoid it. When a child is throwing up, and has large ketones, and high blood sugars, it usually means a trip to the hospital. Ketoacidosis is happening... and only an IV will help. If nothing is done for a while... she could go into a coma and die. I would avoid this. We were going to flush those ketones. I checked her again and finally she was in the 200's. The ketones were moderate.

She drank more fluids. Her little body was coming through this. We were flushing them out. Four and a half hours had passed while we fought those ketones, but we did it! I checked her again and she was 194, high for some people, but in our range. We checked ketones. They were gone. Had it really been the beginning of ketoacidosis? Was she just excited? Was she sick with some four-hour stomach flu even though no one else was sick? Why? Is this how she handles excitement? I know some people throw up when they are excited or nervous, and they don't have diabetes. Was this all in my imagination?

She was fine. She and her sister ran around packing last minute stuffed animals into their rolling suitcase. Blood sugars continued to be fine and the ketones stayed gone.... We flew off to grandma's house.
Now, I just feel so alone. Not even my mom can understand the emotions and fears I felt today. Did I prevent a trip to the hospital with my expert care and assessment of the situation? Was there really even a situation? Will it happen again? Will we ever have to go the hospital to treat ketoacidosis? Ahhh, the questions need to stop.

We will just live each day at a time. We will not search for answers that are not there, but we will be prepared. We will fight this thing. We will make it.

Paranoia

Spring 2001

After dinner one evening, our guests asked if they could check their blood sugar. I think everyone has a bit of a hypochondriac in them, I know I do. We changed the lancet and did a finger poke on everyone. All of the numbers were fine except our one-year-old baby, Katarina. Her blood sugar was 235. I flipped out.

What did this mean? Normal, I've been told, is 70-120. This was over 200. I couldn't have two kids with diabetes. I know I had said once that it might be easier if they both had it; then we could treat them the same, but I didn't mean it. I was barely handling one child with diabetes.

I kept checking her that night and we made an appointment the next day. We were sure she had diabetes. We went to the hospital. They did the blood tests; her Hemoglobin A1C was low... in the 4's. That was good, but what were these high blood sugars? What was going on? We had just experienced two days of random blood sugars with many over normal.

We got a prescription for needles and insulin and then we went home. I was frustrated. Nothing made sense. I looked at our glucometer over and over. Was it lying to me? Could I even trust the thing? What was the problem?

For some reason, my husband's instincts told us to hold off on the insulin and gather a little bit more data. I tried to make her blood sugar go as high as possible. I stuffed her with marshmallows, chocolate syrup and honey. But she was Ok. Her blood sugar would not go higher than 145. We decided to do random checks in the morning, before she had breakfast. If she was higher than 120 in the morning, then we would have an issue.

No issues developed. No issues with diabetes that is. I discovered that she is hypoglycemic, and wakes up occasionally in the 40's or 50's. Most of the time though, she is in the 70's.

We tried to analyze the events and make some sense out of them... Who checks kids who don't have diabetes anyway? No one besides paranoid mothers of more than one child... one of whom has diabetes. There just aren't many paranoid mother studies out there that I could look to for some assurance. Our endocrinologist even said, "I can't tell you what 'normal' is for a child without diabetes. There just aren't many studies done on kids. "
I had researched all the preventions trials, but she was too young. Besides, would I really want to know that she was going to get diabetes when at that time there was not a whole lot that I could do to prevent it? I just had to chill myself out.

My gut still aches though, thinking that someday she might... but then I stop myself. I have to make a conscious effort to live in the moment. I can trust that I will do my best if... and I will know what to do.

For now, I live today. I have three children, one who happens to have diabetes. I will not let my paranoid brain control us or ruin our moments together. We will live each day as it comes, knowing that we have the skills and the resources to handle whatever is thrown our way.

Insanity

Fall 2000

We've learned that child lock and child proof is relative. We've also learned that the brains of children are far more advanced than we give them credit for. One October day, our three year old, brand new insulin pump-wearer went down for her usual nap. Her preferred napping place, for reasons unknown to us, was her car seat. Our 6 month old was already asleep, so my mom and I were going out for a needed shopping break.

We kissed Elizabeth, took her insulin pump out of its back pack so that it wouldn't dig into her back, double-checked that the child lock was activated, we didn't want her giving herself any insulin, you know, and then we left my husband to take a quiet time in the peaceful house.

As we turned left out of our neighborhood, we received a frantic call from Andy, who is usually a mellow guy. Elizabeth had just given herself 50 units of insulin! He had heard her cry out in pain and ran to see what was up. There she was, pump in hand, crying.

We were home in a flash, loaded in the car and on our way to the hospital while calling 9 1 1 on the cell phone. Andy had already poured a half-gallon of orange juice down her throat, and she threw most up on our way. We arrived at the ER smelling foul and yelling for a glucose IV.

Horror followed as they held her down and inserted the IV... then we waited. I tried to be in control. I had been checking her blood sugar every few minutes the whole ride and I didn't stop once we were in the hospital. I wrote everything down and we made sure we were getting the right help. We called her endocrinologist at Children's Hospital.

Next, Elizabeth and I were strapped onto a stretcher and we jumped into the back of an ambulance for a trip to the Children's ER. I was still checking her every few minutes, and she had never gone below 50. She was never unconscious and was actually enjoying the ride. We arrived at the pediatric ER. I continued to check her. They continued with the glucose IV. She began to stabilize.

Andy, my mom and Katarina soon arrived and we tried to breathe for a few moments. Then we sorted out the events that had led up to this surreal experience. Our little engineer's daughter, her father's child, had taken her pump apart, completely bypassing the child lock feature. She had removed the insulin filled reservoir and had pushed 50 units of insulin into the site on her tummy.

The whole thing was insanity. How could we have guessed that she would do that? We had covered our bases, thought ahead and still... it could have been terrible.

We now think of all the possibilities, regardless of how preposterous they might seem and thus far, no more major stories to share. We are thankful parents, thankful for each and every day survived without a drama.

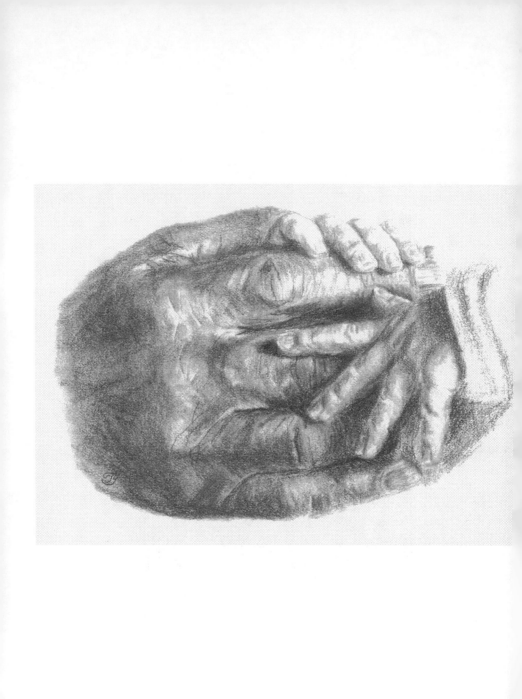

October 12, 2000

One year since our life was turned upside down...

I sit, trying to think back...

One year - what was I doing, where were we...

The doctor's appointment that led to immediate admittance to the hospital, the trip home to get stuff to take to the hospital, the confusion, the unknown, the tears, the pain in our hearts, in her body. Looking around wondering why all these children are here. Cursing the disease that has snatched my child away from me.

The memories - they burn clear in my heart for a few seconds and then they fade, blurred by time. 365 days, countless hours, seconds of life, facing our daily highs and lows, crisis small and large. Sick days, stress, excitement, trouble, fear, joy, love, loss.

How have I managed this year? How have I made it this far without falling into a heap on the floor? I have felt like it, but then what use would I be to anyone lying helpless on the floor?

Somewhere in me, somehow, I have found enough strength to be and to do what I must.

The overwhelming love for my child crutches my emotions and I move on.

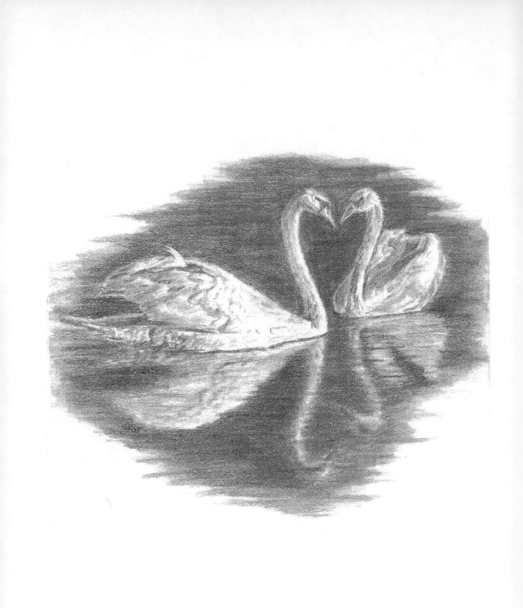

LOVE

I have such an overwhelming desire
to make sure that the love I feel
is shown often.
I want our family to love more than we hate
and laugh more than we cry.

Winter 2000

Daughter –

You have no idea what diabetes really is. You are just three years old. You know that it means - pokes, cranky moods, thirstiness, hunger, anger, tears, smiles, carbohydrates, set changes, shots, a back pack, a pump, doctor's visits, and insulin (whatever that is?).

You do not know that I think about it all the time, or maybe you do, but you just don't know how to tell me yet. You do not know that without good control your life will be full of complications, sickness and even death.

Daughter, I love you. I love you more than I can even believe. I gave you life, gave you a chance to live. I am sorry that along with the life you have, diabetes became a part of you. I wish that I could take it away, relieve you of your disease, and take it myself. I wish that you could be perfect, whole, and free of any worry.

Daughter, I cannot free you from your fate. I cannot cure you. I cannot take away your pain.

Daughter, I can teach you how to live life to the fullest regardless of your disease. I can teach you to be strong no matter what you face. I can teach you by showing you. I bear the burden of your disease now. You are three, you are enjoying life, you are learning, growing, playing. I am thinking, figuring, worrying. But, I can show you how to live.

Daughter, we cannot control your disease, but together we can stop it from controlling us.

Daughter, you are stronger than the disease that rages in you. You can survive.

I love you, daughter.

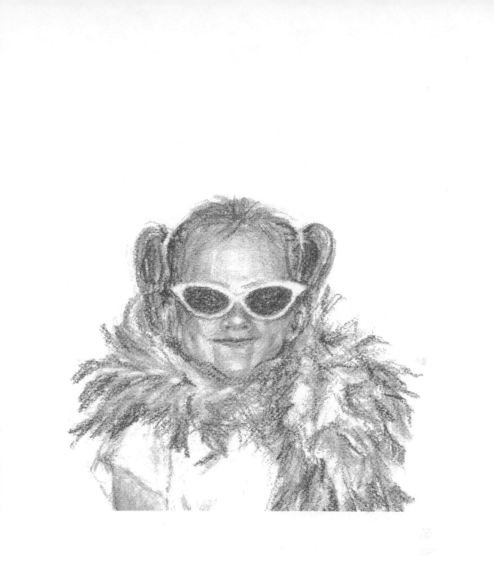

Do I want all my kids to be little molds of each other?
Who are really little molds of me (and my husband)?

    Am I an egotist?
    Am I a conformist?
    Am I a perfectionist?

Do I really think that equality and conformity is good and necessary?

Maybe...
    I don't want to treat one child differently.
    I would like one of them to look like me.
    I don't want to think that one child is better.
    I don't want one to have a disease.
    I want a peaceful family with harmony floating through our walls.

But...
Having everything the same will not bring contentment or peace.
I have three children.
They are as different as they can possibly be and still have come from the same parents.

    One has platinum hair.
        One has strawberry blonde hair.
            One has light brown hair.
    One is pink.
        One is yellow.
            One is white.
    One has diabetes.
        One has hypoglycemia.
            One has no health issues.

So...

I will enjoy the treasures each child brings to our home.
I will not wish for them to be the same.
I will not allow their differences to be a wedge.
I will enjoy my children.
I will give each one the love and attention they need.

I will love them as they are.

DECISIONS

Each day is a constant trip in decision-making. Some decisions are earth shattering, others are inconsequential.

We do our best to research all the possibilities, look at all angles and not close our minds to what might seem a little different or scary.

Do we continue with insulin shots? Do we try an insulin pump? Do we wear red or black sandals? Do we have one child or three? Do we have cheerios or cornflakes? Do we fight hard everyday or do we give up in tears?

We trust that we will make the right choices and if not, we will choose differently tomorrow.

Fall 2000

We didn't think we would ever find a routine after our lives had been turned upside down by checking blood sugar and giving insulin shots, but we made it. We became comfortable with the pokes and the shots. We counted to 3 in various languages as we gave our daughter her daily dose. A few months into our new life, we became concerned that her arms were being used too much. After finally getting into a routine giving her shots only in her arm, we decided it was time to give the tummy and legs a try. But try as we might, there was no budging her from "arms only!"

This new challenge of site rotation seemed daunting. How could we possibly get her to try a new place? I thought back to my childhood, my mom, and the songs she sang to me in stressful situations. I remembered that there wasn't anything a good song wouldn't fix.

Somehow, as I thought of arms - tummy - legs... the little song "sugar in the morning, sugar in the evening, sugar at suppertime; be my little sugar and love me all the time" came to me. Our song of comfort was born. I sang it to my husband, Andrew - "arm in the morning, tummy at supper, leg at bedtime; be my little darlin' and love me all the time"- he liked it. We tried it out on Elizabeth. She loved it and loved singing it with us while we gave her a shot. There's nothing a little song won't fix. She became so reliant on the song that when we would mention it was shot time, she would start singing.

There are days when I wish I didn't have to think about diabetes... Didn't have to be creative... Didn't have to face another challenge. But I get over it as the songs my mom sang to me float through my head, and then I sing to my little girl.

Fall 2000

I want control. All of us do to some extent, but I really want control! Not control over my husband, or my life, or the weather, No, those things don't get to me. I want control over my daughter's diabetes. I want to control it!

After Elizabeth was diagnosed at 2 years and 2 months old, I discovered how much of a control freak I could be. She has been poked more times than a pincushion. I was a wreck if she was low. I was angry if she was high. I was, in short, going nuts. We had gone from two to four shots in less than six months. How do you explain that to a two year old? I had a new baby and a strict dietary schedule was almost ruining me. Insulin shots work, they are a great way to control diabetes, but.... I needed a better way.

One fine abnormal day, I was reading the American Diabetes Association's Diabetes Forecast magazine, which I love to read, but hate to relate to. I need to know the latest and the best. I must be on top of this disease. There was an article about a 5-year-old boy who had gone on the insulin pump. I was thrilled. I had found the answer to my control issues. I was so moved by what the mother had written. I kept nodding my head in agreement. I didn't know someone else felt that way.

To make a long story short, I got in touch that very day with our insurance company to see what amount they would cover. They sent the paperwork, which I returned. Our insurance would cover 100% of the pump, 80% of the supplies. I was on a roll. Next I called her doctor to see what he thought. Fortunately, we have a very progressive doctor who works with us and who wants the best for us. He said, "Why not?"

There was the system to go through first. The meetings with umpteen people to see if we were the right type of family. Screenings to make sure we were committed. I was chomping at the bit, literally foaming at the mouth thinking of what good control we would have. My husband was more cautious, looking at all the angles, all the pros, and all the cons. We balance each other I guess. Finally the go-ahead came. We were set.

Much happened from the time the "Yes" came to the actual putting on of the pump. I wore one (using saline) to see how it felt. My hopes and excitement faded a little as I came down from the clouds. I sat, palms sweating, forehead dripping, teeth clenched, skin pinched in anticipation, a nervous wreck, trying to put the set in me for the first time. Could I really do this to my kid? Could I insert an inch long needle under her skin and then pull it out with the plastic tube still inside her? No, maybe not... but then the control thing came back, yes, yes, we need absolute control. My child will not have complications.

And so we began. I have never worked so hard, been so involved or so emotionally drained as I was the first three months of her being a pump user. Control was nowhere. A three year old requires very little insulin, especially when they are still in a honeymoon and even less on a pump. So, insulin dilution was necessary. We had to fine-tune basal rates, bolus amounts and her carb-to-insulin ratio.

In my control-freakishness, I checked her every 2 hours. Some could scream, "How can you do that?" and I would scream right back, "How can I not?". I am protecting her, assuring her a future free of complications, pain and...

I was an exhausted, nervous, emotional case, much in need of a break, some assurance, something. One day it stopped. I let go. I calmed down. I relinquished control. Her blood sugars have been more stable ever since. Her doctor says she is fairly well controlled.

The moral of this story is: I cannot control my daughter's diabetes. The more I try, the worse it gets. If I stress, she feels the stress, and stress does strange things to a body....

So regardless of shots or insulin pump therapy, the answer is the same. Do the best you can do and let go of the rest.

January 2000

The American family has 1.5 children. We had two girls. Beautiful and amazing. Our hearts were full, but there was this nagging feeling to have one more. We didn't want one more just to have a boy, or to have 3 girls, we just felt the need to have one more. I certainly never imagined myself the mother of three, but there I was, feeling the desire to add one more child to our family.

One more child?

One more chance to have diabetes again?

One more child to think about, worry about, fear for.

One more child to love, enjoy, hold, dream with, teach and learn from.

We listed the pros and cons. We got very technical and involved the right and left sides of our brain. Could we afford another child, would we handle another child, blah, blah, blah, what if, maybe no, could be... enough. The mind and heart often disagree.

We thought that we could provide a good home for a third child.

Ultimately, we decided that diabetes or the possibility of diabetes would not make the choice for us. We knew that we will not allow diabetes to make us regret our choices.

We now have three wonderful children, Elizabeth, Katarina and Jonathan. We cannot imagine life without them.

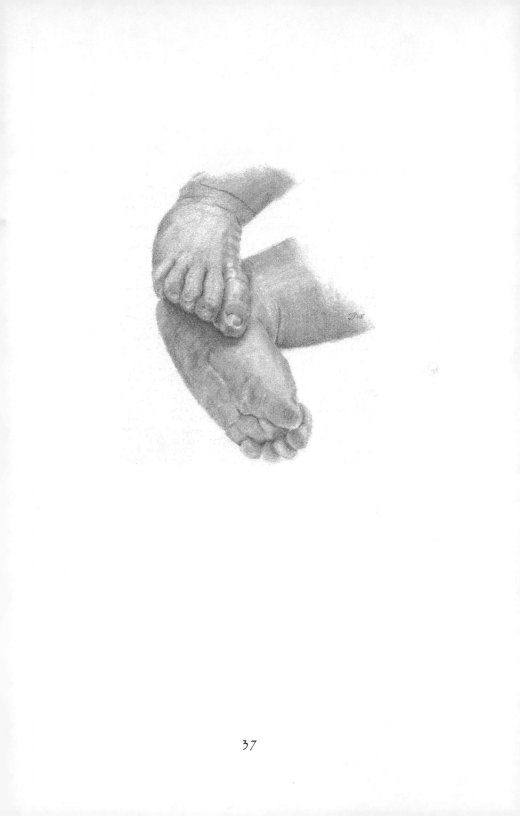

EDUCATION

I can't quite count the times that someone has told me, rather than asked, "She will grow out of this." I cringe, bite my tongue and smile. "No, she has type I or juvenile diabetes, so she can't grow out of it." Then I put on my educator face and launch out on a mini-mission to enlighten this person.

"Juvenile diabetes, Type I diabetes and also called diabetes mellitus, is an auto-immune disease, which means that a part of the body decides to attack itself. At the onset of juvenile diabetes, the islets cells of the pancreas are destroyed. These are the cells that produce insulin. We need insulin to use the sugars we get from our food, to live. This destruction process can take many years, but most of the victims are children."

At this point, the person I am enlightening is looking a little overwhelmed. I continue my mission, undaunted.

"There are many theories as to why this disease begins, but no one can tell you exactly. It is a combination of things; the environment, genetics, a virus or chemical, extreme stress to the body and who knows what else needs to happen for the disease to begin its work. Every parent can tell you what they think caused the disease. There is no conclusive evidence yet to say for sure... although researchers are getting very close. Once the disease begins to work, the body is never the same. At some point, the islet cells quit producing insulin completely and without intervention the body will die."

Now my poor victim is totally overwhelmed, so I take a different approach and share what else I usually hear about diabetes.

"Most everyone we know knows someone with diabetes; their grandparents, or aunt or uncle or one of their parents. They take a pill and can control it with diet and exercise. It is usually in the family for generations. They have

Type II diabetes, which is not the same disease."

They smile in agreement, thinking of their own great aunt.

"Well, diet and exercise will not prevent diabetes in my child. It is not caused because she is overweight. It is not hereditary, although we have three cousins affected by the disease in our family. The right genes need to be present, along with some other factors, but type I is not passed down through the generations."

"Juvenile diabetes usually comes out of nowhere and smacks families in the face and heart."

I stop talking. My mission is complete. I walk away; my feet placed solidly in front of me, and I leave my friend with a spinning head.

ADVICE TO MYSELF

1) Do the best I can possibly do for my child.

2) Love her more than I can ever imagine loving someone.

3) Don't look past the FACE to get TO diabetes.

4) Learn to let go and accept that there are things in life that are uncontrollable. Learn how to make those things as tame as possible.

5) Try not to make diabetes the ONLY thing that identifies Elizabeth.

6) Be a BETTER example myself. Life is not going to magically change because we have to have a more defined schedule.

7) Be more consistent in food preparation, carb counting, insulin coverage.

8) Make sure to breathe. If I don't take care of myself, I can't take care of anyone else.

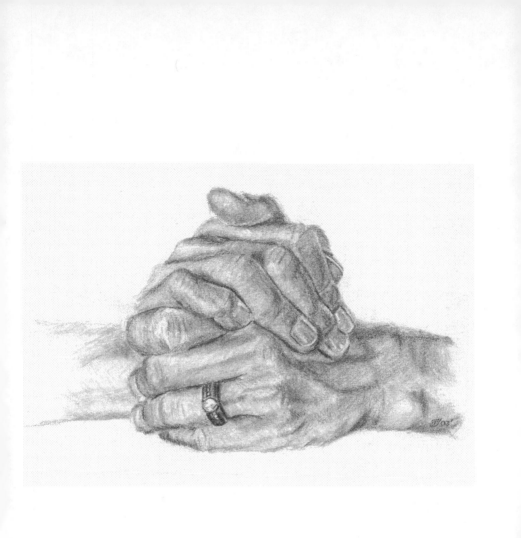

I put on my rose-colored glasses
occasionally.
I sit down with them on
and
look around.

What I like about my child having diabetes:
1. that I know what it is
2. that it will help us be more scheduled
3. we have met so many wonderful people
4. not much really... today.

What I like about my child:
1. sparkling eyes
2. curiosity
3. humor
4. laugh
5. kisses
6. hugs
7. tummy
8. round cheeks
9. eyelashes
10. love
11. questions
12. art
13. play
14. imagination
15. style
16. and on and on and on and on.

I am learning to trust myself; trust that I am doing my very best.
Part of my very best is not allowing Elizabeth to be just
'Diabetes Must Control',
but rather
Elizabeth,
my daughter who happens to have diabetes.

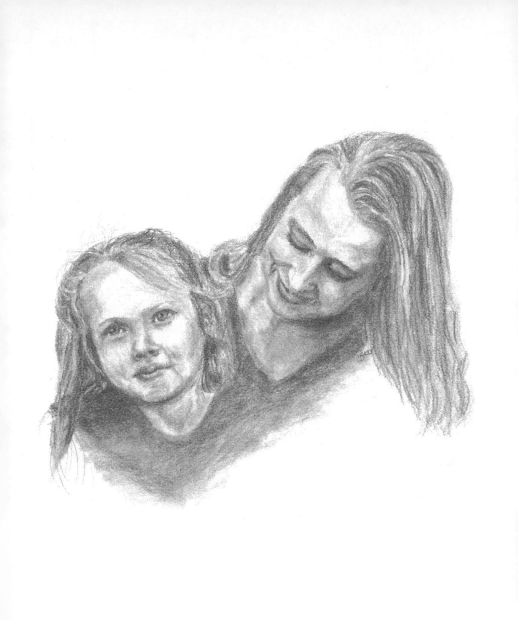

A DIFFERENCE

As I became more involved with diabetes and finding resources to help us, we came across JDRF. The Juvenile Diabetes Research Foundation is a fundraising organization founded by parents, with money raised going directly to research for a cure to diabetes. I was hooked. I had found a place where I could make a positive difference and be a good example to Elizabeth. I can show her that we can each make a difference if we get involved. Our contribution is important, no matter how large or small.

JDRF holds a Walk to Cure Diabetes every year. We have enjoyed forming a family team with some of our friends and making a difference together. We send out a letter each year to family and friends. We have been amazed by their support, not just with the money they send back, but the notes of encouragement as well. We have learned that given a chance to help, many people are more than willing. Together we all make a difference.

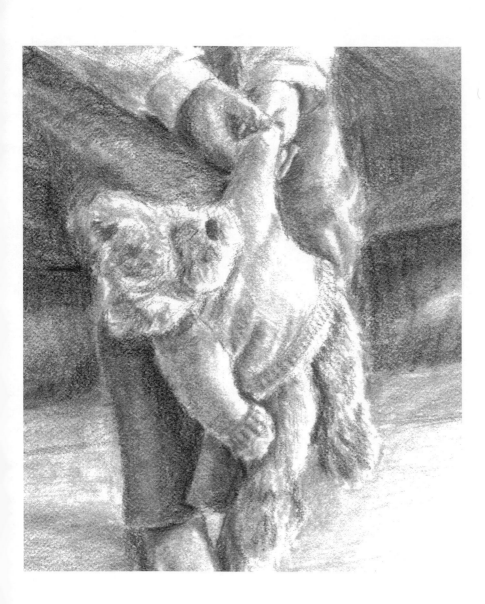

Spring 2001

Imagine for a moment the total chaos of emotions. Mainly, how do we explain to this innocent child that she must get a finger poke 6-8 times a day, 1-2 times at night and have 3-4 shots a day? How do we deal with the fact that her body is destroying a part of itself? How do we accept that this disease could kill her?

We were ignorant as to the complexity of this disease, what it means, what it was, what it can do. All we knew was that it meant shots and no sugar. During the 3 days that we were in the hospital, we were immersed in classes. We learned all about diet (things are not as drastic as they used to be, just much awareness and a lot of carbohydrate counting), about the disease itself, how to do a finger poke, and how to give shots (we practiced on ourselves). Then we went home. Home was not the same.

There has been a lot we have learned since returning home with a child with special health care needs (i.e., a disease that takes an enormous amount of energy, both physical and emotional, to control). We could have sat back and said, "ok, here we are; we'll do the minimum amount required to keep her alive." But No Way! We made a pact to do everything we could to keep her disease in control. We could not and cannot stand by and let this disease ravage her body. Dealing with diabetes is a 24/7 job. There are no breaks, no slack time, no ' let's forget about it for today.' The truth is, if I am not vigilant, if I do not count her carbohydrates, if I do not give her the insulin she needs, she will die.

Insulin is not a cure. Insulin keeps her alive.

Spring 2002

The other day, as I was preparing to change Elizabeth's pump site, she said to me,
"Mom, let's get money to buy that medicine to take away my diabetes."
I wanted to say,
"Ok, here's $5.00, let's go down to the store and get it for you. You've had this disease long enough."

For now though, I can only wish for that 'medicine'. Elizabeth is a preschooler, so we spend a good portion of our days in a fantasyland. Most of the time I am the wicked stepmother and she is Cinderella doing 'all the cooking, cleaning, scrubbing and mending (I wish?).

Soon, fantasy will become a reality –
not the wicked stepmother bit, but a cure!

Spring 2003

I was poking around Elizabeth's brain last week, trying to get in her head to see how she feels about her life and about having diabetes. Life is still fairly simple. She is sure that her dad goes to work to make money for her piggy bank. She thinks she is rich with $26.00 and being in school is fun, especially P.E.

I asked her what she dislikes most about having diabetes. She came up with the most obvious things such as pokes, site changes, and not getting to eat everything she wants, when she wants it.

I also asked her what she liked about diabetes. "Well", she said, "I like lows because I can have sugar. And I like highs because I can have cheese and pickles." Pretty simple.

A few minutes later, she was playing in the living room and she said, "Mom, I just remembered, the thing I don't like most about having diabetes is that if I didn't have a poker, or a pump, or insulin, I would die."

Well, if there is a more compelling reason to get out and raise money for a cure, I haven't found it: A five year old, innocent in so many ways, yet completely aware of her own mortality because she has diabetes.

"Elizabeth, we forgot to do a poke again... argh! How can we forget sometimes especially when..." - "Yeah mom, when it is something I have to do the rest of my life. Why don't we go on the Walk to Cure today?!! Then they will find it today! And I won't do pokes... and set changes and....What do you think a cure looks like!?! I think it will be in a little cup and I will drink it."

I wish I could have made up this little exchange of words between my daughter and I. I wish that this was a little letter I was writing for someone I knew... someone who we would like to help. Then, I could step away and let go of it. I wish that I could find that little cup of cure myself and pass it around. I know too many children and adults who need it....

I have a child with diabetes. I have a cousin Lance with diabetes. I also have a cousin Lisa whose son Noah has diabetes. I have another cousin Tom, who has diabetes. I have friends – Rhonda, Jan, Georgia, Mary Alice, Vanessa, Zuraya, Kathy, Mike, Dave, Michelle, Susan, Kim, Lori, Peni, Nancy, Eric, and Bernadette whose children have diabetes. My friends- Gail and her sister, Kerry, Sarah, Ted, Joe, Judy, John, Chrissy and Dave have diabetes. I have friends- Chris, Melinda, James and Jim who have siblings with diabetes. Our mail carrier lost a spouse to juvenile diabetes.

There are more... friends and acquaintances. Every day it seems that I meet someone else who is affected by diabetes.

ENOUGH

STRUGGLE

Sometimes I look around
Sometimes I just look down
Some days I look to heaven
Sometimes I don't look at all.

I know others around me suffer
some even fall
I feel the pain of everyone
and I do nothing.

Sometimes I am angry
Sometimes I just spit
Some days I am empty
Sometimes I can't feel a thing.

I know my family is suffering
some never let it show
I feel the pain so intensely
and I can do nothing at all.

Sometimes I am too busy
Sometimes I am stuck in myself
Some days I can't handle anything
Sometimes I come back.

I know that I should get over this
some days are so long
I feel the pain as I move on
and I begin work on myself.

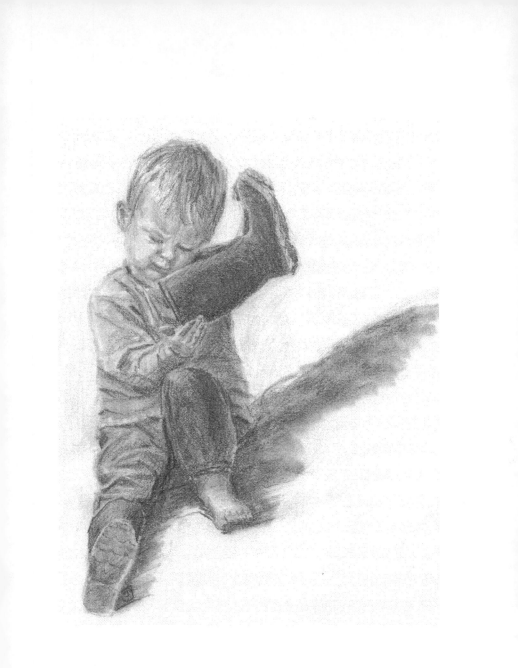

Everyday

I must plan for weeks if I am to be away from my child for a day. I must send a grocery store and a user's manual with her. I must also attach a GPS device to myself, so that her care-giver (who is quite a rare find), will know my every move and how to reach me.

I must plan eighteen years ahead now that my child is going to school. We hear advertisements all the time for college funds and starting early. "Plan ahead", they advise.

I am planning ahead, but I have an HCP plan (signed, health care provider form) ten pages of detailed documents, a five day disaster kit and emergency preparedness supplies, a box of low blood sugar supplies, a daily blood sugar log, a child- care manual (complete with a picture of her on the front), low and high blood sugar charts for every room that she might venture into, two glucometers, test strips, batteries, alcohol swabs. Have I forgotten anything?

I cannot send my darling growing girl to school with a kiss and say, "have a good day, we'll see you when you get home." No, I must plan for carbohydrate intake at lunch, snacks, recess, PE, surprise birthday cupcakes, ice cream day, tests, germs and what else. I must make sure the teachers, PE instructor, librarian, music director, office and recess staff, principal, guest teachers, nurse, and janitors are all on the same page. They all need 'training' to be aware of the signs and symptoms, the possibilities, the necessities, the reality of diabetes.

I get dizzy. I get mad. Why should we all have to bear this burden? Mainly, why does she have to bear this burden, this juvenile diabetes curse that has snatched away her carefree childhood?

There is no answer to that question, I know that. I just wish there was. So, as is our style, we do more than the minimum. We prepare for everything and we smile.

Diabetes is a struggle, but we won't let it ruin her life.

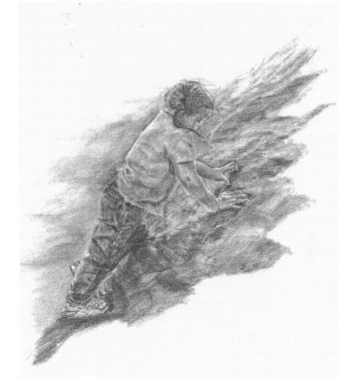

The years go by
as a blink and an eternity
bound up in an insulin vial.

Fear. Insanity.
Growth. Hope. Security.
Comfort. Loss. Grief. Pain. Anger.
Love. Joy. Determination.

Our feelings cycle through the stages
as we pass through time.

We mourn not just once,
the life lost to this disease.

But we accept the joys brought
and the depth gained
because of our struggle.

Waking up high -
fighting to get into control -
falling out -
going too low -
rebounding past the sky and
plateauing in the clouds for awhile-
Finally going to bed half-way decent
only to wake up at 2 am
to find her in the clouds again
get her down -
check her an hour later -
Finally -
which we've said six times already
finally we're in range...
Finally I can sleep.

How crazy it is to have a perfect day of blood sugars
followed by an outrageous day.
It is so hard not to let these outrageous days define our life.

Tonight I struggled with perfection.

No, not that I have achieved perfection, not even close, but with the fact that perfection is what I want and there is no way we will have it. Perfection, as in normal blood sugars all the time. We may have normal blood sugars some of the time, but never all of the time.

I have a hard time with this.

I must understand and accept that IMPERFECTION is what diabetes IS and that is how it will be always.

I will learn to accept that imperfection does not mean I, or my child, have failed. It does not mean that I am bad, wrong, stupid, not scheduled enough, not strict enough, can't count, don't care...

It means that diabetes is.

I feel lost without my disease.

When I am out with my other kids, and I don't have to check blood sugars, watch what they eat, or give insulin, I feel guilty.

It is so much easier without diabetes. I forget that having a child with diabetes, or having diabetes is a big deal because I am so focused on making it not a big deal.

My job now is to acknowledge my guilt, validate it and let go.

I have no choice.

RESOLVE

I was listening to the radio-a-thon for a cancer research center as my kids and I were driving home yesterday. I was crying to myself as I listened to the stories of parents who had lost a child. Every time the announcers asked for someone to call, I wanted to. My daughter in the back seat, who has a daily fight of her own with diabetes, started asking questions. "What is it, why are you crying, where do they live?" The announcer said it one more time, please call now and help. Elizabeth yelled to me from the back, "Call Now, Mom, I want to help kids with cancer." I did call and pledge because we know that a lot of little bits make a lot.

It is easy to get wrapped up in our struggle with diabetes. I feel so angry sometimes that it is in our family. Through our experiences we have learned that it isn't what the struggle _is_ that matters; it is what is produced as a result. If having diabetes in our family is going to help me and my children to see the pain and suffering of others, and if it is going to give us the tools to care, to love and to want to help, then bring it on. We can stand it.

My thoughts and prayers go to every family that has some type of disease raging through their house. The diseases have their differences, some are more devastating than others, but we can support each other. We hope for a cure to everything. In the mean time, we will live today and make a difference... even with a smile, or a call to an organization that brings hope.

I don't want to get stuck asking
the questions that cannot be answered.

At some point the wrong things happened at the right time...
to me, my child, an immune system... and now there is diabetes.

It is here to stay...

WE WILL DO THE BEST WE CAN TODAY.

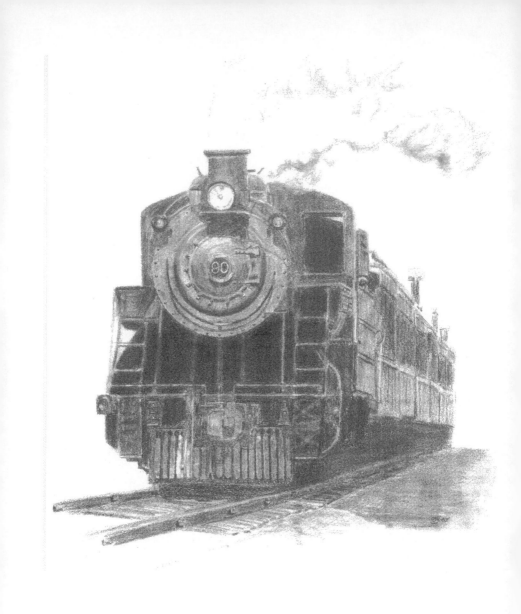

We will not cower in the face of diabetes.

If we cower, what do we teach our child,
who must live her life with the realities of this disease?

Do we want to teach her, that she shouldn't do what she feels in her heart
because of the possibilities of something happening?
No.

We will teach her to think clearly, act wisely and live fully.

Diabetes is just a part of us
like a shoe

comfortable for now

soon

we will be ready soon
to kick it off

and

trade it for a cure.

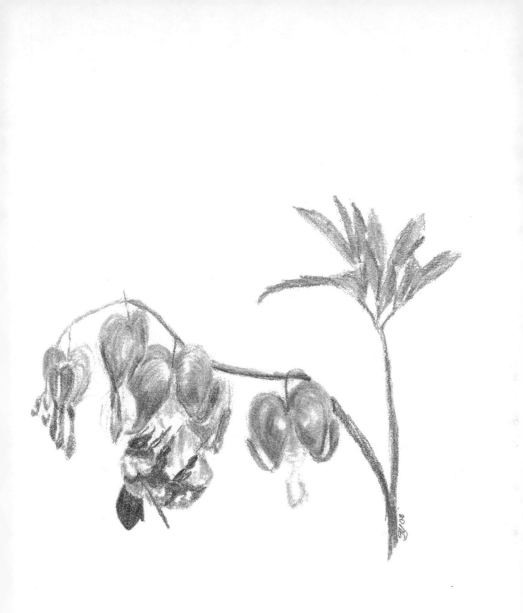

Someday I will pass this disease on to her.
She will think about it more often than not.
She will check herself always, do site changes, drive herself to the doctor...
Live...

and I will not know what to do.

I am teaching her how best to take care of herself,
by taking care of her... now...

Someday I will learn from her how she just lived.

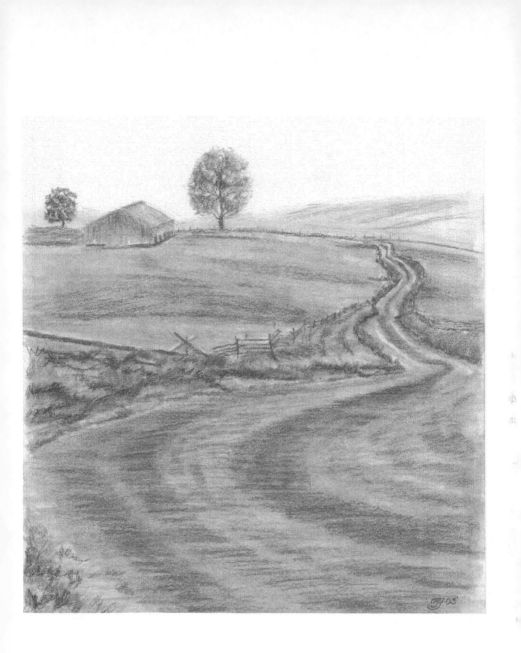

THE JOURNEY

Fall 2003 and into the future...

Elizabeth is 6 years old.
Every day she reports to me how much bigger she is.
I have many more years of writing.

Tomorrow she will leave home.
She will take with her whatever we have managed to pass on to her.

Good luck, daughter.
I am always with you.

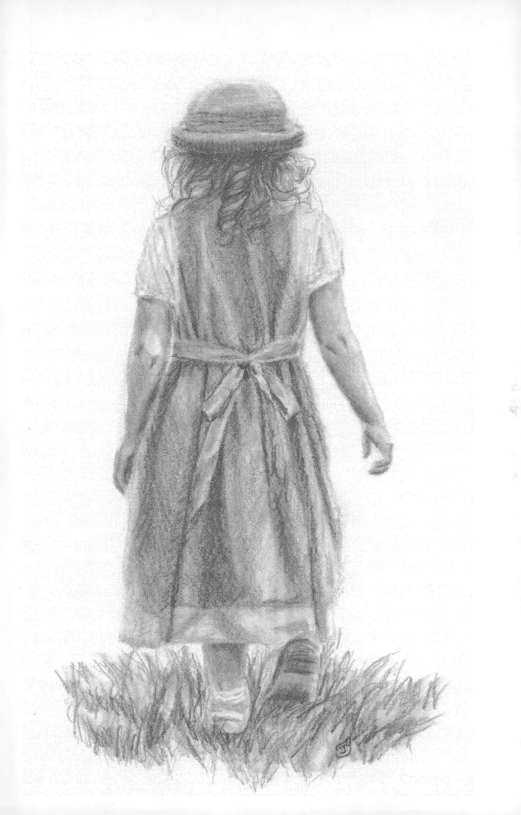

TERMS AND DEFINITIONS
- as told to a 6 year old -

Abnormal blood sugar: A blood sugar over 120 when no food has been eaten for a long period of time. A blood sugar over 200 two hours after eating food. These numbers are different from person to person.

ADA: American Diabetes Association. An organization dedicated to education and research of adult onset diabetes or Type II Diabetes and Juvenile Diabetes or type I diabetes.

Autoimmune disease: A disease in which the body attacks a part of itself.

Basal rates: The twenty-four hour 'base' rate that has been programmed into the insulin pump. The basal rate covers the amount of sugar that the body produces naturally.

Blood sugar: The amount of sugar in the blood. It is also called blood glucose level.

Bolus amounts: The equivalent of an insulin shot. It is given by the insulin pump and covers the carbohydrates eaten at a meal.

Carbohydrates: Food that contains sugars and starches. They provide a quick and sure source of energy to the body.

Carb-insulin ratio: A number that tells how much insulin is needed for every gram of carbohydrate eaten.

Checking blood sugar: The blood sugar level is checked by doing a finger poke and then placing a drop of blood on a test strip in a glucometer.

Diabetes Mellitus: Another name for juvenile diabetes or type I diabetes.

Finger pokes/pokes: A tiny lancet, or little needle, is used to poke the finger to get a drop of blood to check the sugar level.

Glucagon: A special shot that is used to bring a body out of an unconscious insulin reaction. It is also a hormone that helps the body release stored sugar.

Glucometer: The machine used to check the blood sugar levels.

Hemoglobin A1C: A blood test used to measure the amount of protein in the blood. It is like a report card for parents. A good range for kids with diabetes is between 7% and 8%.

Highs or Hyperglycemia: Too many sugars running around the blood stream. The blood sugar level is above normal.

Honeymoon period: The time after diabetes diagnosis, where the body is still producing a little bit of insulin. This period varies from a few weeks to a few years.

Insulin: A hormone produced in the pancreas, which allows sugars to be used properly by the body.

Insulin dilution: Mixing insulin with saline to use in an insulin pump. This may be necessary so that the correct amount of insulin can be given.

Insulin pump: A little device that allows the insulin to be given steadily.

Insulin reaction: Way too much insulin is running around the body. This term is used interchangeably with hypoglycemia. Sometimes seizures and unconsciousness occur.

JDRF: Juvenile Diabetes Research Foundation. A fundraising organization founded by parents in the 1970's. It is the leading contributor to research for a cure to juvenile or type I diabetes.

Juvenile Diabetes: Another name for type 1 diabetes or Diabetes Mellitus. Most people diagnosed with juvenile diabetes are children, but it can attack a body until its late 30's or early 40's.

Ketoacidosis: Not enough insulin is available to cover the amount of sugars in the body so the blood sugars become very high. Vomiting, lethargy and nausea occur because too many toxins are running around the blood stream. These toxins cannot find a way out, so they build up. Without treatment involving fluids and more insulin, the body will go into a coma and eventually die.

Ketones: A build up of sugar in the urine because of high blood sugars or sickness. There has not been enough insulin in the body for a long time so the sugars have no place to go. Ketones are measured as trace, small, moderate or large. Large ketones can be very dangerous and lead to hospitalization.

Lows: Hypoglycemia. Too much insulin is running around the body. The blood sugar level is below normal.

Medicine: A five year olds definition of a cure.

Normal blood sugar: Typically in adults, this means a blood sugar reading between 70 and 120. There are no conclusive studies as to what 'normal' is in children although it is probably similar.

Saline: A clear, harmless, sterile fluid that can be mixed with insulin. It can be used to practice giving shots and can be used in an insulin pump trial.

Set/site: A set is a catheter-like, plastic tube that is inserted into the fatty area of the stomach, upper bottom, or leg. It is connected to an angel hair pasta-sized tube that is hooked to a reservoir of insulin that is placed in the insulin pump.

Site changes and rotation: The plastic piece that is inserted into the body is changed every few days. Site rotation is moving around the places on the body where a shot or set change is done.

Shots: A method used to give insulin.

Type I Diabetes: An autoimmune disease in which the body attacks the cells that produce insulin. It cannot be prevented or managed without insulin.

Type II Diabetes: A disease in which the body is unable to use the insulin that it produces. It can be prevented and managed with diet, exercise, pills and insulin.

Walk to Cure: An organized walk that happens in many locations throughout the world. It is sponsored by the JDRF. Funds raised at the walk go directly to research for a cure.

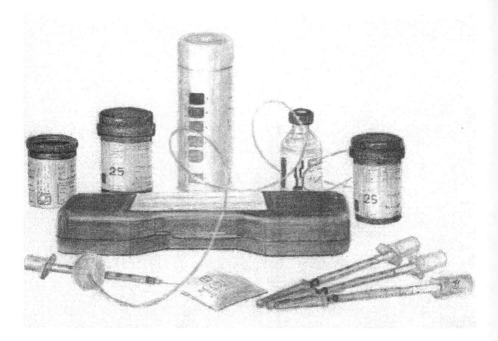

A cure for diabetes is closer than ever before. Islet cell transplants, and artificial pancreases on the horizon, prevention trials, gene discoveries, new and more efficient insulin, new devices for controlling diabetes and so much more that gives us hope. Every month something new is announced.

This is an exciting time because we know that in our lifetime diabetes will become a disease of the past.

Many, many thanks to my dear friends
for their help throughout this never- ending, book-making journey.

Editors:
Sara, Loren, John, Michelle, John, Becky, Jeanine, Brian,
Vicki, Susan, Gwen and Lori

Production Manager:
Andrew

Illustrations:
Jeanne and Becky

Creative Advice:
John at www.inkcogneato.com

Medical Review:
Gail

Encouragement:
Ruth, Marvin, Rhonda, Jo, Linda, Allison,
Kerry, Jill, Katarina, and Jonathan

Inspiration:
Elizabeth

A portion from the sale of each book, up to $5.00, is donated
to organizations dedicated to curing childhood diseases.
For more information visit
www.zaypub.com

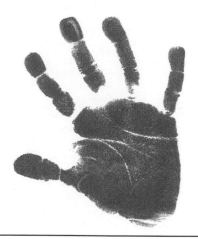

Elizabeth Jo Zosel

THANK YOU FOR READING THIS BOOK.
I hope that our journey will be a help to you.

Made in the USA
Lexington, KY
30 May 2015